HOMESTEAD COOKING:
Food Preservation Basics

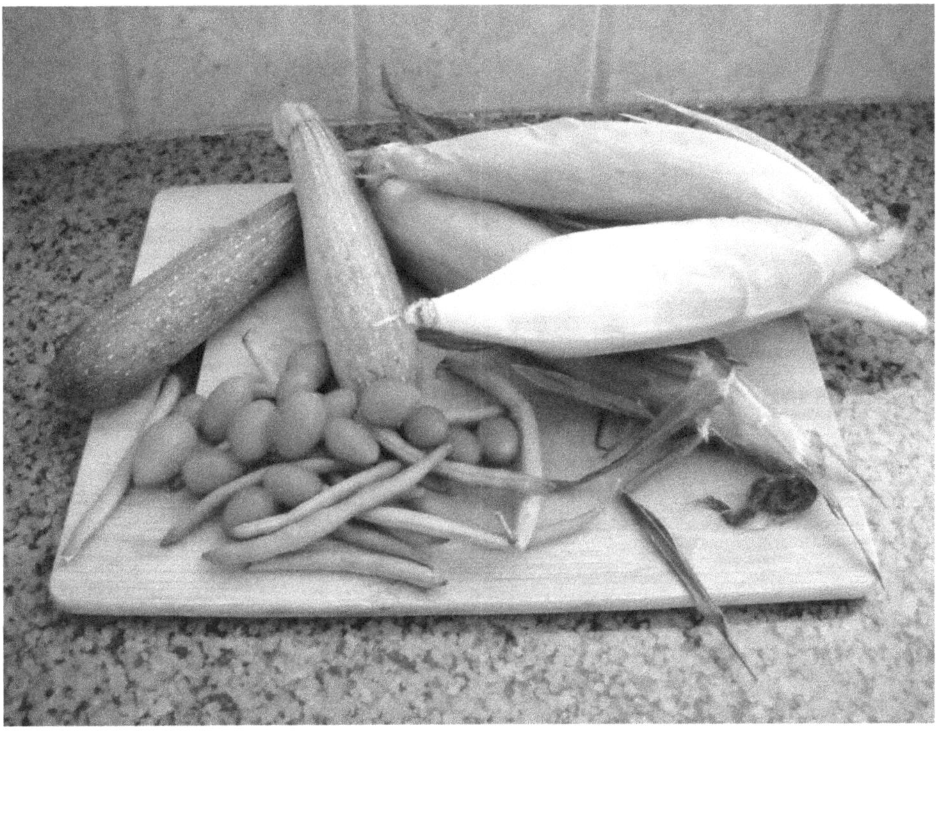

Table of Contents

INTRODUCTION

In my humble opinion, you haven't lived until you've tasted a homemade pickle. Store bought pale in comparison to these crisp, green spears of pickled heaven (sorry Vlasic!). My husband claims he hates pickles; he routinely picks them off his hamburgers and deli sandwiches when we eat out. Yet, I can't keep him away from my home-canned pickles. And, believe me I've tried…but, he's found all my best hiding spots.

The same goes for canning home-grown tomatoes or freezing fresh garden-grown corn. The taste of home preserved produce far outshines the tinned and frozen vegetables you'll find in the grocery store. In fact, the taste of home preserved produce outshines the *fresh* produce you'll find in the grocery store.

Canning and freezing your garden vegetables lets you enjoy the taste of summer produce year around. I know food preservation sounds intimidating, especially canning, but don't let it scare you. This easy-to-follow guide will have you happily and safely canning your tomatoes and freezing your green beans in no time. Once you've read this book you'll know:

- What equipment you need to start canning and freezing your produce (Chapter 1).
- How to safely preserve food (Chapter 2).
- Which food preservation practices you should avoid and why (Chapter 2).
- How to calculate canning processing times at high altitude (Chapter 2).
- How to easily blanch vegetables for freezing (Chapter 3).
- What "blanching" is and why it's important (Chapter 3).
- Why you should use bottled lemon juice instead of fresh for canning (Chapter 4).
- How you can easily remove the skins from tomatoes for canning (Chapter 4).
- Why exhausting your pressure canner is important, even if you're using a self-venting canner (Chapter 5).
- Why pressure canning, in many respects, is actually better and easier than water bath canning and freezing (Chapter 5).

The information in this guide is presented in an easy to follow and straight-forward manner. I try to avoid using jargon as much as possible. For jargon that must be used, I've provided clear, simple definitions in the first chapter that you can refer back to as necessary. Chapters are broken into clearly labeled sections with step-by-step directions. While this short guide prevents me from including a lot of canning recipes, when appropriate, I provide times, tips, and tricks for freezing and canning various types of vegetables.

By the time you're done reading this guide, you'll be hiding your delicious, home canned pickles from your significant other. FYI, empty canners make a great place to hide things… pickles, M&Ms, Mrs. Field's cookies, whatever your guilty pleasure.

I'm not here to judge.

CHAPTER 1

FOOD PRESERVATION 101:
BASIC TERMS AND DEFINITIONS

Your garden produced a bumper crop. You have tomatoes, beans, corn, peas, and cucumbers galore. You eat zucchini at every meal, including breakfast. Your coworkers run and hide when they see you coming at them with bags of fresh greens. You hate to see your home grown produce go to waste; you expended a lot time and effort growing it. But, you're running out of recipe ideas, and there's a limit to the amount of vegetables you can get your kids to eat. You passed it two weeks ago when your broccoli crop came in.

So, why not try canning and freezing your extra produce? That way, the vegetables stay fresh, and you can enjoy your vine-ripened crops all winter long.

I can already feel the anxiety building at that suggestion. Food preservation, especially canning, seems to make even the most seasoned vegetable gardeners nervous. Visions of food spoilage and death by botulism swarm, and gardeners make their peace with crops rotting on their kitchen counters rather than chance it happening in their pantries and freezers. However, a little know-how will help allay your food preservation fears and get you canning and freezing your vegetables like the Jolly Green Giant.

Spoilage is caused by microorganisms (enzymes, mold, yeast, and bacteria) feasting on our food. It's just Nature's way of telling us the food is no longer fit for human consumption. Canning and freezing, however, interrupt the food spoilage cycle, as microorganisms can't survive temperatures that are too hot (above boiling) or too cold (below freezing). To safely preserve food, you just need to make sure your vegetables reach the right temperature levels when you're canning and freezing your produce. In essence, that's all there really is to it. Simple, right?

I can sense that you aren't entirely convinced. You're still thinking food preservation sounds more complicated than that. But, that's just because, like every activity, canning and freezing has its own lingo. Composting and plant thinning were probably new concepts when you started your vegetable patch, but now you garden like a pro, and neighbors routinely request a batch of your compost that makes plants grow like magic.

Learning a few canning and freezing terms and their definitions will help alleviate some of your food preservation fears and give you the confidence to can and freeze your produce.

■ **Blanching**
Submerging vegetables in boiling water for a short time prior to freezing. Blanching better preserves vegetable flavor, color, and vitamin content.

■ **Canner**
Large cooking-pot style container used to process (boil) canning jars. Canners are bottom-lined with a shallow rack to keep jars off the heat source and prevent breakage. Types of canners include water-bath canners, pressure canners, or hybrid varieties than can be used for both water-bath and pressure canning.

■ **Canning Jars**
Thick, glass jars approved for canning use, such as Mason, Ball, or Kerr jars. Canning jars generally come quart-sized and pint-sized, although some other odd sizes are available (half-pint, pint-and-a-half, etc.).

Jars are also available with a wide mouth or narrow mouth. I recommend wide mouth for packing vegetables (easier to get your hand in and out of the jar) and narrow mouth for canning sauces and salsas (easier to fit a funnel for pouring).

Jars can be reused. But, be sure to check jars for cracks and chips, especially around the jar's rim. Discard any with defects as these jars will not properly seal.

■ **Cold Pack**
Placing raw vegetables into the jars and then filling the jars with hot brine or liquid prior to processing. Vegetables are cold-packed to help preserve crispness.

Pressure canned vegetables are usually cold-packed.

- **Fingertip Tight**
  You'll often be instructed to tighten the jar's screw bands "fingertip tight." Screw on bands using your fingers, giving an extra twist with your *fingertips only* once the band stops. Do not use any tools or the full force of your grip to tighten bands.

- **Headspace**
  The amount of empty space between the rim of the jar and the vegetables you're canning. Most canning recipes call for a headspace of ½" to 1".

- **High Acid Vegetables**
  Vegetables, like tomatoes, that have a pH value of 4.6 or lower. High acid vegetables can be water-bath canned. Vegetables that are mixed with a vinegar-based brine or solution, like pickles and sauerkraut, are also considered high acid and can be water-bath canned.

  High acid vegetables do not freeze well and are better canned.

- **Hot Pack**
  Vegetables are simmered in boiling brine or liquid prior to being added to jars and processed. Vegetables are hot packed to remove the air from vegetables, leading to less shrinkage during processing, and better sealing.

  Water-bathed vegetables are often hot-packed.

- **Lids**
  The metal lid sits atop the canning jar and contains a compound that will vacuum seal the lid to the jar after processing. Canning lids are disposable and, unlike the jars and bands, can only be used once, and must be replaced each time you can.

- **Low Acid Vegetables**
  Vegetables that have a pH value higher than 4.6. Most vegetables fall into this category. Low acid vegetables must be pressure canned. If you still have a fear of pressure canning after this tutorial, know that low acid vegetables do freeze well.

- **Pressure Canning**
  A style of canning that uses steam pressure to process vegetables at temperatures of 240°, a temperature at which bacteria cannot exist. Low acid vegetables must be pressure canned as their acidic content is not high enough to kill bacteria.

- **Processing**
  Boiling vegetable-packed jars in the canner. Different vegetables will require being processed for different lengths of time.

- **Reprocessing**
  If jars do not seal within twenty-four hours of processing, the contents can be reprocessed in a sterile jar with a different lid. Reprocessing can leave the produce mushy and unpalatable. Rather than reprocess, you can opt to refrigerate unsealed jars and use the produce as you would when you first open a sealed jar.

- **Screw Bands**
  The metal band or ring that screws on to the canning jar. Screw bands keep the jar lids in place while the canning jar is processing.

  Bands can be reused as long as they still adhere well to the jar and are not rusted or bent out of shape.

- **Sealing**
  The air-tight lock that forms between the rim of the jar and the metal lid. The metal lid contains a rubber-like sealing compound that will affix to the canning jar as it cools after being processed. You'll hear a "ping" once your lid seals.

- **Water Bath Canning**
  Submerging jars in boiling water, so that jars are covered by at least an inch of water. Jars are then boiled for the recommended time (depending on produce being canned) to kill all microorganisms. Water bath canning reaches temperatures of 212° and is appropriate for high acid foods.

As you've probably guessed from the list of definitions, canning vegetables takes a little more equipment than freezing vegetables. For freezing vegetables, you just need a large pot of boiling water, a large bowl of ice water, and containers to hold your frozen produce. The list of canning equipment is a bit lengthier though well worth the investment, as some produce, like tomatoes, can't be frozen but are delicious canned.

Canning Equipment List

- Canner...I recommend a hybrid variety that can be used for both water bath and pressure canning.

- Canning Rack...most canners come with a canning rack.

- Canning Jars with Bands and Lids...these are sold in flats of a dozen. If someone has bequeathed you a number of canning jars, you can buy replacement bands and lids.

- Funnel...canning funnels with openings designed to match canning jars work best.

- Jar and Lid Lifters...will save you burning your fingers or dropping your jars while using regular kitchen tongs. I speak from experience.

CHAPTER 2

AVOIDING CONTAMINATION: BEST FOOD SAFETY PRACTICES

Having read the first chapter, I'm sure you're feeling much more confident about freezing and canning your produce. As well you should. The basic process is much easier than you've likely been led to believe. However, that being said, taking measures to ensure food safety is critically important when preserving produce, and you should make every effort to preserve your vegetables in the safest manner possible.

The danger of food contaminates shouldn't leave you so fearful that you avoid canning and freezing, but you do need to be aware of the best, and current, food safety practices. While you great-grandmother may have canned food using the open kettle method (hot-packing produce and using the heat of the canned product to create the canning jar's seal) and lived to tell the tale, open kettle canning is largely discouraged now as the foods canned by this method don't reach high enough temperatures to kill microorganisms. Other canning methods to avoid include:

- **Open Kettle Canning**
  Yep, I just mentioned this one, but lots of people still insist on canning this way. Please don't be tempted. I can understand the enticement of open kettle canning as you can skip a step and not boil your jars, but you're at a much higher risk of your canned goods spouting bacteria. And, while you think you may be able to tell if food is spoiled, that's not always the case (more on that in a second), and you risk serious illness if contaminated food is ingested.

- **Steam Canning**
  A steam canner uses (you guessed it!) circulating steam to seal canning jars. Yes, this may sound a lot like a pressure canner; however, a pressure canner keeps steam trapped in the device, guaranteeing that your vegetables reach an acceptable temperature level to safely preserve your food as well as creating high levels of pressure to vacuum seal your jars.

  Not so with a steam canner. The temperature of the circulating steam can't be guaranteed, relies on heat rather than pressure to seal the jars, and steam alone doesn't create enough heat to kill any microorganisms lurking in your vegetables the way steam and boiling water do.

■ **Paraffin Wax Seals**
This is another canning throw-back from generations past. Usually used for canning jams and jellies, hot paraffin wax would be poured over the canned product to create the jar's seal.

Unfortunately, the seal can't be guaranteed until the paraffin wax is removed later prior to consuming the product. If the jelly looked okay, it would be spread on toast (and we know why that's a bad idea based on your new knowledge of open kettle canning). If the jam was growing mold, as it did about half the time, the jar would be tossed. A waste of time and effort that would have been better spent boiling jam-filled jars to create a proper seal.

■ **Upside Down Sealing**
I've never seen this done, but I'm told this is how some people can in Europe. But, don't let the European tag fool you. This is more akin to Great Britain's food or Spain's finances than British soccer or Spanish tapas. The essence of this method is that food is hot-packed, and the cans are turned upside down, relying on heat and gravity to seal the jars.

Just like the open-kettle method, the jars are not boiled, so the canned produce doesn't reach hot enough temperatures to ensure all microorganisms have been killed. Add to this that the jar lids can become warped from being flipped the wrong way, and you're practically guaranteed an unsafe seal if the jars even seal at all.

■ **Oven and/or Solar Method**
This is just what it sounds like. Food is hot-packed into jars, and the jars are placed in the oven or outside in a sunny area. The heat from the oven or sun seals the jars. Again, the food never reaches boiling temperatures, so the food is really not safe to consume given that microorganisms may have survived this lackluster canning process.

Ditto for using a microwave oven to can, a grill to can, or even, a dishwasher to can (yes, I've actually heard of people doing this).

In addition to using a pressure canner or water-bath canner (and only using a water-bath canner for high-acid produce) to properly preserve your vegetables, you should also be sure to:

- **Sterilize all canning jars before use.**
  To sterilize your canning jars, wash them in hot, soapy water (including lids and bands). Then, boil the jars for fifteen minutes. Use a pot large enough that the jars will be completely covered when they're standing upright. Remove the jars with clean, sanitized tongs and set the upright jars on a clean towel.

  Sanitize rings, lids, and canning utensils in a similar fashion. Though, be wary about boiling lids as this can affect the rubber seal. Instead, after jars have boiled for fifteen minutes, turn off the heat source, and then add lids to the pot. They can remain in the hot water for up to an hour.

- **Blanche all vegetables before freezing.**
  In addition to better preserving vegetable crispness, color, and taste, blanching kills any bacteria that are hanging out on your produce. And, while freezing slows bacterial growth, those little microorganisms can reactivate when produce is defrosted.

- **Can and freeze produce when it's at its freshest.**
  Not only will you get a better preserved product, you'll reduce the risk of food spoilage and food-borne bacteria and illnesses.

- **If you live at high altitude, know that you will need to process canning jars longer.**
  Follow high altitude cooking and canning guidelines for your area. General rule of thumb is increase water-bath processing time 1 minute for every 1,000 feet above sea level if total processing time is less than 20 minutes. If processing time is more than 20 minutes, increase time by 2 minutes for every 1,000 feet.

For pressure canners, increase pressure to 11½ pounds for altitudes between 2,000 and 3,000 feet. Increase pressure by ½ pound for every 1,000 feet thereafter.

■ **Reprocess all jars that have not sealed within twenty-four hours**
Change the lid and use a freshly sanitized jar. If you don't want to reprocess your produce, either refrigerate the jar immediately or discard the contents.

■ **Never used canned produce that you suspect is contaminated.**
Discard jars that have cracked, unsealed, or those whose lids are leaking or bulging. If the produce develops mold or an odd smell, toss it. If the contents of a jar foam or spurt when the lid is opened, don't use them.

Trust your gut instinct: if something about the canned produce seems off, throw it out. Better to be safe than sorry, sick, and nauseous.

So, what do you risk if you cheat and skip a few steps during canning? Not to scare you…well, maybe to concern you enough to stick to our accepted, safe canning plan…, but:

■ **Botulism**
This is the one that terrifies all new canners, as botulism is not really detectable through sight, smell, or taste, and one little bite of botulism-contaminated food can be fatal. The good news is that botulism spores can't survive the high 240° heat of a pressure canner, so as long as you're pressure canning your low-acid produce, you're safe.

Botulism is also fairly rare. Only about a hundred cases were reported in the United States in the last decade. But, one-third of those cases were attributed to improperly home-canned food. All the more incentive to follow best canning practices at all times. If you're nervous about botulism, pressure can. Even high acid vegetables, like tomatoes, can be pressured canned for ultimate peace of mind.

While botulism is certainly at the extreme end of food-borne illnesses, we all know that even the most mild cases of food poisoning are not fun. You may be a little tired of hearing this, but always follow up-to-date, best food preservation practices to avoid food spoilage and food-borne illnesses.

Fully indoctrinated as to food safety? Great! Now you're ready to move on to freezing produce and drying herbs.

Chapter 3

Freezing & Drying:
The Lighter Side of Food Preservation

If canning still worries you, start your foray into food preservation by freezing your produce. Freezing is a quick, beginner-friendly method of food preservation that requires little equipment. Just a large pot for boiling water and large bowl for holding ice water along with a few plastic bags or containers that are freezer-friendly. Consider:

- Most low acid vegetables, like corn, peas, beans, carrots, broccoli, and okra, freeze well.

- Soups also freeze well, so for a quick meal option, you can make large batches of soups, broths, or vegetable stocks, and freeze several smaller portions for later use.

- High acid vegetables, like tomatoes, along with sweet potatoes and squash don't generally freeze well raw. But, if these produce items are cooked beforehand, they can be frozen with better results.

Before freezing, most vegetables should be blanched. I say *most* because, like all things, there are exceptions to every rule. These rule-bending vegetables include:

- **Onions and Peppers (Sweet or Bell)**
  Onions and peppers can be sliced or chopped and frozen without blanching.

- **Chile Peppers (Anaheim, Poblano, Jalapeño, etc.)**
  Like bell peppers, chiles can be frozen without blanching. However, most recipes call for these peppers to be peeled. For convenience sake, it's far easier (and tastier) to peel peppers before freezing.

  Roast the peppers on a grill or under a broiler until the skins begin to brown and blister (5 to 20 minutes, depending on pepper size). Remove the chiles from heat and place them in a sealed container for 10 minutes. This will loosen the skins and make them easy to remove.

  Peel the skins and remove the stems and seeds. If you're roasting and peeling a large batch of chiles, wear disposable gloves (your hands will appreciate this gesture). You can either freeze the peppers whole and chop them into smaller sizes.

■ **Beets**
Beets should be cooked until tender, and then frozen, either whole or sliced.

■ **Potatoes (including sweet), Winter Squash, & Pumpkins**
These produce items should be cooked through and mashed prior to freezing. If you're freezing a soup or stew, don't include potatoes in the batch, as frozen potatoes get watery and leak. Instead, add potatoes when the soup or stew is defrosted, prior to eating.

■ **Mushrooms**
Mushrooms should be sautéed before they're frozen. Mushrooms can be frozen either whole or sliced.

■ **Tomatoes**
Tomatoes are really best canned, but if you must freeze them, peel tomatoes and remove stems and seeds. To easily peel a tomato, dip the tomato in boiling water for 30 seconds to loosen the skin. Stew the tomatoes in a large pot until tender (10-20 minutes should do it) and transfer to a freezer-safe container.

Frozen tomatoes are best used in sauces, soups, and stews.

All other vegetables should be blanched prior to freezing. Blanching helps preserve the vegetables' flavor, color, and taste as well as helping kill microorganisms prior to freezing. To blanch and freeze your produce:

1. First, you're going to prepare your vegetables just as would if you were cooking them for dinner. Wash your veggies in cold water and chop them into the sizes you plan on using them in later. For best results, freeze vegetables at their height of freshness, right after they're picked.

2. Bring a gallon of water to a rolling boil in a large pot. Also, have a large bowl of ice water standing ready.

3. Submerge the vegetables in the boiling water for 2-5 minutes per the chart below and cover the pot. For simplicity and to avoid having a bunch of loose vegetables bobbing around in the water, place your vegetables in a covered wire strainer or cheesecloth bag. If you don't have a wire strainer or cheesecloth bag, be prepared to fish your vegetables out with a slotted spoon.

4. After scalding the vegetables for the requisite amount of time, remove them from the pot and plunge them into your waiting bowl of ice water to stop the vegetables cooking. Leave them in the ice water for the same amount of time as they spent boiling.

5. Drain the vegetables and pat them dry. Make sure no liquid makes it into the freezer containers as this can cause ice crystals to form on the produce.

6. Pack the vegetables into their freezer bags or containers and put them in the freezer. You're done!

Blanching Times

Shelled Beans and Peas:	1-3 minutes, depending on size (1 minute small legumes, 2 minutes medium legumes, 3 minutes large legumes)
Green or Snap Beans:	3 minutes
Soy Beans:	5 minutes
Broccoli:	3 minutes (for 1½" stems and pieces)
Corn (cobs):	6-8 minutes, depending on size
Corn (whole kernel):	4 minutes
Okra:	3-4 minutes, depending on size

Carrots:	2 minutes (1"-2" pieces, skins removed)
Zucchini:	3 minutes (½" slices)
Cauliflower:	2 minutes (1" pieces)

If you're freezing multiple batches of the same vegetable, you can use the same pot of boiling water to continue blanching. If you're switching vegetables, use a fresh pot of boiling water.

Since frozen vegetables have been blanched (thus partially cooked) prior to freezing, they require shorter cooking times than they would if they were fresh. Adjust cooking times for frozen vegetables accordingly.

Some vegetables just can't be frozen. Radishes, salad greens, celery and scallions won't freeze. Nor will cucumbers (although they can be canned as pickles). You'll have to eat them when they're picked or pass them off to a grateful neighbor. Ungrateful neighbors can also be used during high harvest times when you have a lot of available produce.

Herbs are another garden product that can't be frozen. However, herbs can be dried. For example:

- If you have a dehydrator, herbs can be dried in 1-4 hours on a heat setting of 95°-115°.

- If you don't own a dehydrator, you can still dry herbs. Tender leaf herbs, like basil and oregano, have to be dried quickly to avoid spouting mold. If you live in a low humidity area, dry tender leaf herbs, in small bunches, hanging, in brown paper bags. Punch a few holes in the sides of the bag to allow for air circulation.

  If you live in a high humidity area, dry tender leaf herbs individually on paper towels in a cool oven. Separate the leaves from the stems and lay the leaves (not touching) on the paper towel and cover with another paper towel. Leave the herbs in an oven, overnight, with the oven light on.

- Less tender herbs, like thyme and sage, can be tied in small bundles, and hung upside down to dry. Dry herbs indoors for better flavor retention.

Herbs are finished drying when the leaves crumble easily. Store dried herbs in airtight bottles or containers.

CHAPTER 4

WATER BATH CANNING:
TOMATOES AND PICKLES AND SALSAS, OH MY!

Hooray! You've taken the plunge and decided to can. Water bath canning may seem less intimidating than pressure canning, and it's a great place to begin. Plus, while you may be able to get away with freezing corn and beans, tomatoes, a stock crop of most gardens, just do not hold up well in a freezer. But, due to their high acidity content, tomatoes can be canned via the water bath method.

Canning Tomatoes Using the Water Bath Method

Ingredients
- Tomatoes (20 pounds of tomatoes will net you about 7 quart jars canned, or figure 7-8 large tomatoes per quart jar)
- Bottled Lemon Juice or Citric Acid (will be used to increase acidity content of jars)
- Salt
- Water (& lots of it....you'll be using water to fill jars, sanitize jars, and process jars)

Equipment
- Water Bath Canner with Canning Rack
- Wide-Mouth Quart or Pint Canning Jars with Lids and Bands
- Funnel
- Jar and Lid Lifters
- Several Pots (for boiling water, tomatoes, jars, band, & lids)
- Kettle (not entirely necessary, but I find it helpful for keeping a constant supply of boiling water flowing)
- Clean Towels (to set sealed jars on)
- Clean, Damp Kitchen Cloth or Wash Rag (for wiping rims of jars)
- Tomato Corer (again, not necessary but useful)
- Sharp Knife & Cutting Board

1. Start boiling water. You're going to find that canning requires a lot of boiling water.

   Fill the canner halfway with water and begin heating, keeping the canner covered. For hot-packed food, the water needs to be preheated to 140°; for raw-packed food, the water needs to be preheated to 180°. The jars will need to be covered by 1"-2" of water when they're placed in the canner. You might find that you need to add additional water to the canner once the jars are in place, so keep a kettle or an additional pot of boiling water nearby.

   Jars, bands, and lids will need to be sanitized in another large pot of boiling water according to the directions in Chapter 2.

Also bring a third, medium sized pot of water to a boil. This pot will be used to remove the skins from the tomatoes.

2. Wash all tomatoes. Be sure to select fruit that is firm and as fresh from the vine as possible. Avoid using old or wilted tomatoes, and never can tomatoes from vines that have died (either from disease or frost). Green tomatoes have an even higher acidity content that ripened tomatoes, and can be safely canned.

   The tomatoes' skins need to be removed as they become tough and chewy after canning. Plunge the tomatoes into boiling water for 30-45 seconds (no more than a minute!). The tomato skins will then loosen and can be easily removed. For even easier skin removal (and to spare your fingers a few burns), submerge the tomatoes briefly in cold water after they've been boiled.

3. Remove skins. If canning tomatoes whole, remove the core. Or, halve or quarter tomatoes, as you prefer.

   If you're canning a particularly juicy variety of tomatoes, like Early Girls, consider removing some of the tomatoes' seeds and juice, so you're canning more tomato meat rather than just juice. If you have the time and patience, removing the seeds and juice from any tomato will give you a meatier canned product.

   Cut away any bruises or dark spots on the tomatoes. Also remove any tough areas around the stem and core.

4. Place tomatoes in jars, leaving a ½" of headspace.

   Add 2 tablespoons of bottled lemon juice or ½ teaspoon of citric acid per quart jar (use 1 tablespoon of bottled lemon juice or ¼ teaspoon of citric acid per pint jar). Be sure to use *bottled* lemon juice rather than fresh as the acidity content of the bottled lemon juice is more uniform.

If desired, add 1 teaspoon of salt to each quart (or ½ teaspoon to each pint).

Add hot water to jars, keeping a ½" of headspace. Use a canning funnel to add the water to avoid splashing any of the jar's contents onto the jar's rim.

5. Run the handle of a wooden spoon or flat plastic utensil around the inside of the jar to remove any air bubbles. Don't use a metal utensil, like a knife.

Gently wipe the rim of the jars with a clean, dampened cloth to remove any spillage. If the rim of the jar has any food particles on it, the lid won't form a good seal.

Place the lids on the jars and screw on the bands, fingertip-tight (snug, but not over-tight).

6. Place the jars on the canning rack, inside the canner. The canning rack will keep the jars from touching the bottom which could cause them to break. Also make sure the jars aren't touching the canner's sides or each other.

Make sure the jars are covered by at least 1" of water; 2" of water would be even better. Additional boiling water can be added to the canner during processing time to keep the water level constant, but pour the water around the jars, not on them.

Keep the canner covered while processing. Make sure the water maintains a complete boil while the jars are being processed. If the water stops boiling for any reason, raise the burner's temperature and return the water to a vigorous boil. You'll also need to start the jars' processing clock over again. Sorry!

Process quarts for 45 minutes and pints for 40 minutes. If you live at higher altitudes, adjust processing time accordingly (see Chapter 2).

7. Once the jars have processed, turn off the heat and remove the canner's lid. Let the jars sit for five minutes before removing from the canner with a clean jar lifter.

Place the jars on a clean towel in a draft-free area. Keep the jars at least an inch apart from each other. Let the jars cool for 12-24 hours. They've been through quite an ordeal, so try not to disturb them. No pressing on the lids yet!

After the jars have cooled, you can check to verify they've sealed. Gently press the center of each lid. If the lid is permanently depressed, your jar has sealed!

If the lid pops up and down, unfortunately, the jar has not sealed. Don't worry about it; it happens to everyone. You have two choices: you can either reprocess the jar, using a new lid and sanitized jar, or you can refrigerate the jar and use the contents as you would for any newly opened can of produce.

Water Bath Canning Other Products

The process for canning other high-acid products, like tomato sauces, salsas, or pickles will be mostly the same as canning tomatoes. Processing times and packing methods may differ, but you'll still sanitize your jars, fill them leaving a ½" of headspace, remove bubbles, process jars evenly spaced in a canner, and allow jars to cool and set for 12-24 hours. There are a lot of recipes out there for canning tomato sauce, spaghetti sauces, pickles and sauerkraut, and salsas. Just a few things to keep in mind during your canning experiments:

- Only use recipes that have been approved for canning. Canning recipes will have a calibrated acidity content that will keep your canned food from spoiling.

- Some recipes call for vinegar rather than bottled lemon juice or citric acid, especially pickles. Vinegar works to increase acidity content just like lemon juice and citric acid do.

- When following a recipe for salsa or marina sauce, be wary of adding extra herbs and spices as these extra ingredients can lower the acidity content of the jar.

- If in doubt, pressure can your jars. The elevated temperature of a pressure canner will keep your food safe. You can also pressure can your tomatoes for additional peace of mind. Also know that pressure canning requires shorter processing times, so your canned goods will retain better color and flavor using this canning method.

  Wait… you don't know how to pressure can? Well, let's move on, then, to Chapter 5.

CHAPTER 5

BUILDING STEAM:
INTRODUCTION TO PRESSURE CANNING

Now that you've tried water bath canning, you're thinking that pressure canning can't be that much different. And, you're right! The basics of sanitizing your jars and preparing and packing your produce are the same. The method of processing your jars, however, is going to change.

I know I've mentioned this before, but for safety's sake, I'm going to mention it again. All low acid vegetables, which basically means all vegetables except tomatoes, must be pressure canned. The microorganisms that cause food spoilage and dreaded botulism poisoning can survive boiling water, which only reaches a temperature of 212°. Tomatoes can be canned via this method because their acidity content is high enough that the acid, in addition to the heat of the water bath canner, keeps microorganisms in check.

Not so for corn, beans, peas, carrots, and other low acid vegetables. Produce with a low acidity content needs to be processed at the 240° a pressure canner can guarantee. And, if you're thinking that you'll just add a lot of citric acid or lemon juice to your peas before processing them in your water bath canner, that won't work (nice try, though). You're going to have to make your peace with pressure canning.

And, you should. There are a lot of advantages to pressure canning. You can be assured that your jars (if properly sealed) are safe since they've been processed at such a high temperature that no nasty bacteria will survive to ruin your canned goods. And, when you pressure can, your produce will be processed for far less time than they would be in a water bath canner (5-15 minutes versus 45-60). Shorter processing times means better produce. Vegetables that are pressure canned have more flavor, better texture, and better color. Also, you should know that though you can water bath can your tomatoes, that doesn't prevent you from pressure canning them with the same taste results as other pressure canned vegetables.

Pressure canning does require a special piece of equipment in the form of a pressure canner: a large pot with a locking lid, pressure gauge, pressure regulator, and air vent. The cover locks in place and seals to allow heat and pressure to build inside the canner, so that ideal 240° processing temperature can be reached. Different vegetables will be processed at different pounds of pressure (usually 11), and processing time begins once the canner's dial reaches that amount of pressure.

Every pressure canner comes with slightly different directions, so always follow manufacture guidelines. In general, however, when you use a pressure canner, you will:

1. Fill the canner with 2"-3" of hot water (about 3 quarts, depending on the size of your canner). To keep your jars from getting water-stained, you can also add 2 tablespoons of white vinegar to the water in the canner. Just like with water bath canning, you'll need to use a canning rack on the bottom of the canner.
   Place your jars, filled with veggies, lids and bands in place, into the canner. Also, just like water bath canning, the jars shouldn't be touching the sides of the canner or each other.

2. Place the cover on your canner and lock the lid in place. Make sure the vent pipe is open. Turn your stove on high and begin heating your canner. Use a level burner as a tilted burner can mess with the pressure regulator.

3. Bring the water in the canner to a boil. You want a steady flow of steam moving through the vent pipe. Once you have a steady flow of steam, you'll need to "exhaust" your canner. This just means letting the steam flow through the vent pipe for ten minutes.

   Exhausting your canner is very important as it ensures all air is removed from the canner. If air remains inside the canner, the temperature can't reach 240°, so don't be tempted to skip this step. You're already saving processing minutes by pressure canning rather than water bath canning, so you don't need to cut any corners to save a little time. If you have a self-venting canner, I still advise you exhaust it, just to be on the safe side. The method by which vegetables are packed has been shown to affect the air content of a self-venting canner.

4. Close the vent pipe. This is accomplished in different ways depending on the canner. On mine, I just place the pressure regulator over the vent pipe. The canner will begin to build pressure. This happens fairly quickly, so keep a close eye on the pressure gauge.

5. Once your canner reaches the correct amount of pressure (usually 11 pounds, but varies depending on recipe and altitude), start your processing timer. Watch the pressure gauge and adjust the heat to keep a constant amount of pressure. If the pressure keeps building, reduce heat.

   If the pressure dips below what the recipe calls for, turn the heat up to return the canner to the correct pressure. Just like if your water bath canner stops boiling, you'll need to start the processing clock over. Sorry again! But, it's always safer to over-process rather than under-process.

6. Once the jars have processed for the requisite amount of time, turn the heat off. If you're strong, you can move the canner to a cool burner, but pick it up rather than slide it to avoid scratching your stove (again, I speak from experience).

7. UNDER NO CIRCUMSTANCES SHOULD YOU REMOVE THE CANNER LID UNTIL THE PRESSURE HAS COMPLETELY VENTED! Attempting to remove the canner lid before the pressure returns to zero is a good way to get yourself on YouTube when your neighbors film your canner lid goes shooting through your roof. Pressure is funny like that.

   Also, don't rely solely on the pressure gauge to judge if the canner is completely vented. Instead, watch your cover lock and overpressure plug. They will drop once the pressure is reduced. Also, no steam should escape the vent pipe when it's reopened after pressure appears to have been vented.

   After you are absolutely, positively sure pressure has been completely reduced, open the vent pipe and wait ten more minutes.

8. Now, you should be safe to open the canner cover. Lift the lid towards you to avoid getting hit in the face by a cloud of hot steam.

   If the lid sticks at all while you're trying to open it, there still may be pressure inside the canner. Wait a bit longer to open, just to be safe.

9. Lift jars out of the canner with a jar lifter and set on a clean towel to cool, just like you would if the jars had been water bath canned. After 12-24 hours, check jars to verify they've sealed, and you're done.

Congratulations! You have officially pressure canned your produce, and you are now a food preservation extraordinaire! You can also can vegetable stocks and broths in your pressure canner. As with salsas and sauces, be sure to follow recipes that are approved for canning.

CONCLUSION

Well, our time together is ending. I hope you've enjoyed learning the ins-and-outs of food preservation. You're now ready to hot-pack (or cold-pack), process, and seal your canning jars. You know which vegetable you can safely water bath can and why you need to pressure can the rest. You know which veggies you need to blanch before freezing and the few exceptions to the blanching rule. If you didn't understand those last three sentences or were unsure of the answers (or where to find them), you might want to do a quick review. No worries. That's the benefit of having an easy guide to refer back to. Trust me, I review the literature before I start a canning batch all the time.

One last, quick piece of advice. Before the start of each canning season, it's a good idea to have your pressure canner checked to make sure the gauge is still accurate. Most county extension offices offer that service (along with a wealth of canning and food preservation information). If you're not conveniently located to a county extension office, most pressure canning manufacturers have a site you can send your canner to for servicing. The dial gauge can be a little finicky, and if it's off, food safety can be compromised as your canner may not be reaching the pressure it says.

If you're anything like me and it's the start of your garden's harvest, you likely have a counter-full of produce just waiting to be put up. So, I'll leave you to it.

Good luck and happy canning! And, freezing! And, drying!

www.ingramcontent.com/pod-product-compliance
Lightning Source LLC
Chambersburg PA
CBHW070132290526
45789CB00005B/2222